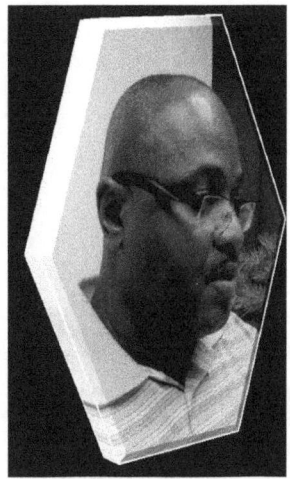

"Scarred for Life"

An inspirational guide to overcome the emotional and physical scars of life!

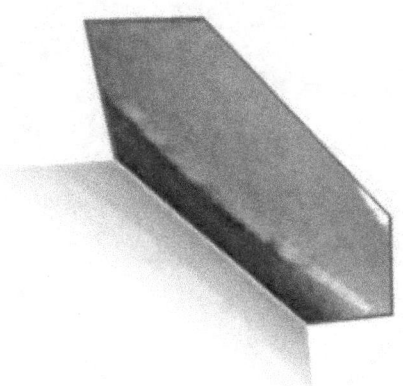

By Sergeant First Class Thaddeus L. Edwards

(United States Army Retired)

Each of us has gone through a storm

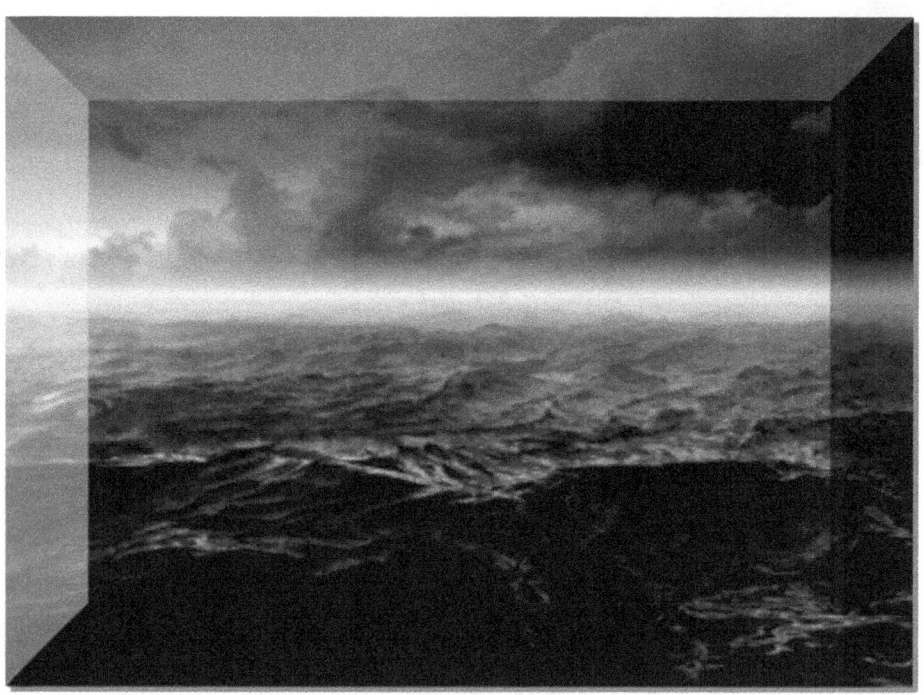

Face your tornado head on

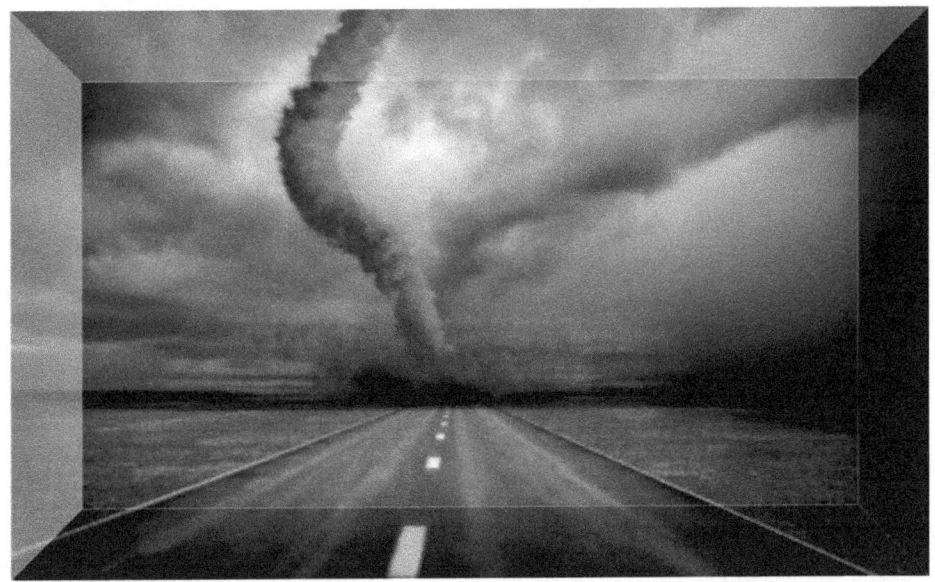

Do you feel like you are scarred for life?

An inspirational guide to overcome the emotional and physical scars of life!

Thaddeus L. Edwards, Sergeant First Class

(United States Army Retired)

Introduction

Scarred for life is true account of the intrinsic and existential events that scarred me both mentally and physically, and how I overcame. It is a story that parallels the life of millions of people only on a different timeline wrinkle in space, and how similar we all are in the end. From the day people are born expectations, hopes, and dreams, are bestowed upon the newest member of the family as a source of hope to erase all past family failures. As a hardened member of society with the ability to see outside what is in the general realm of the social conscience, I am going to show that what has happened will happen, and will happen repeatedly until this planet no longer exists. There are those that commonly believe in humankind, that humanity in general is kind hearted and giving. This may be true in parts of civilization that have not been contaminated with the demon that is life. Hurdles and tests are primary obstacles faced in one's lifetime, but there are inherent and external forces that bombard and upset the natural flow of life throwing it off track until the pendulum can be bought back to its nominal state of balance. People see what they generally want to see through thick-rimmed glasses that block their peripheral vision allowing them to dismiss anything happening around them that does not affect how they go about living out their existence. Perception is not reality, if it were a defendant would be guilty until proven innocent based on perception. A name defines who you are and how people treat you. My name is Thaddeus and I am scarred for life.

"Scarred for Life"

An inspirational guide to overcome the emotional and physical scars of life!

By

Author: Thaddeus L. Edwards

Cover Design by Thaddeus Edwards

Photography by Thaddeus Edwards

Brochure by Thaddeus Edwards

Flyer Design by Thaddeus Edwards

Printed in the United States of America by www.lulu.com

ISBN: 978-0-578-03596-3

First Edition

Published 2009

Published by The 3rd Planet's Ad Spot @ Zyardsale.com, LLC 1963 Belhaven Drive Orange Park, Florida 32065, U.S.A. Copyright © 2009 Thaddeus L. Edwards all right reserved. No part of this publication may be reproduced, stored in a retrieval system, or transmits in any form or any means, electronic, mechanical, recording or otherwise, without the prior written permission of The 3rd Planet's Ad Spot @ Zyardsale.com, LLC http://www.zyardsale.com

About the Author

Sergeant First Class Thaddeus L. Edwards (United States Army Retired) is currently the Chairman and CEO of The 3rd Planet's Ad Spot at Z Yard Sale.com. He is a native of Mobile, Alabama. He graduated from John C. Fremont High School in Los Angeles, California in 1982. Sergeant First Class Retired Thaddeus L. Edwards is a graduate of the University of Phoenix and holds a Diploma from the Logistics Management College.

He served as the Force Integration and Analysis Manager for a 30,000-person installation. In addition, he served as Senior Personnel Management Specialist for over 1500 Person Company. During his twenty-year career, his assignments included Nuremburg, Germany, Fort Benning, Georgia, Athens, Greece, Fort Hood, Texas, Memphis, Tennessee, Fort Richardson, Alaska, Houston, Texas, and Fort Campbell, Kentucky.

Sergeant First Class Retired Edwards's awards include the Bronze Star Medal for combat operations in Iraq, the Meritorious Service Medal, The Army Commendation Medal, and the coveted Pinnacle Award.

Thaddeus is a strong motivational speaker and masterful instructor who has the gift to shed light on the dark. Life is real, and he ensures that you appreciate it!

Scarred for Life

An inspirational guide to overcome the emotional and physical scars of life!

Table of Contents

Scar I   The beginning:........................ 13

Scar II   Lost Childhood:...................... 22

Scar III Social Discomfort:....................28

Scar IV   The Transition:........................33

Scar V   Poignant Moments:.................... 45

Scar VI   The Career:.......................... 62

Scar VII The Foundation:...................... 71

Scar VIII The Dysfunctional Family:..........79

Scar IX   Philosophy of determinism:........ 90

Scar X   Philosophy of rationalism:.......... 94

Conclusion...................................... 122

Appendix A: self-assessment

Appendix B: supplementary information

Acknowledgements

GOD: Special thanks to god our savior. His blessed hand has been with me even when I did not know. He is the only one who never gave up on me. He is the great I AM.

MOM: Mom has been both parents to me. I am so grateful for the guidance and strength you displayed in allowing me to make mistakes and find my way as a man.

WIFE: You have bared many of my scars and have remained strong in Christ even when I was not. You have inspired me for twenty-one years and as much as I complain about this and that, you are my soul mate

Mentor: Nick Trisch played a major role in my development into the civilian sector. Through his guidance and patience, I was able to deprogram from my former career as a soldier to become the CEO of Z Yard Sale.com

Mentor: Linda Billups is my friend. Her refined leadership skills helped me see things in a different light. She taught me how to lead from the heart as well as the mind.

Sons: Thaddeus and Raphael are my legacy. I love them because they are so different from me. I never had a dad. Helping them develop into good men was my responsibility and I hope that I did them both proud as a dad.

Daughter: Brianna, my only daughter is the light of my life. I spoil her, but she deserves it. Her personality and energy brings a bright enthusiasm to the room when she sings.

Colleague: Jeremy Godboldt who I served with on my last assignment and deployed to combat in Iraq with is a true friend. He hails from a family of Army men that fought in Vietnam and on. His uncle was killed in Vietnam, which was depicted in the movie we were soldiers. He still serves and is serving proudly. He always believed that I would do something special.

Scar I

The beginning

It must be nice to have a spoon full of money fed to you at birth, but I was born in a filthy downstairs bathtub in Mobile, Alabama. Early on, the scars came fast and furious like hurricanes out of the Atlantic attacking the Florida coast. My earliest memory was of my stepfather who was an abusive person who got his kicks out of making my three sisters, mom, and I suffer through his crap on a daily basis. In order to punish me, he placed me under an iron bed frame and had me hold it up until I collapsed at the age of four. He then beat my mom in front of us all until she bled from her ears and nose.

The girls of the family Teresa, Tara, Marie, and Tonya were all younger than so I felt obligated even at the age of four to protect them. How can a four year old protect anyone? Well let us see, I had the ability to speak and let him know even at that stage that what was happening was not right. In doing this, it bought his wrath upon me so many times that I developed an introverted personality, unable to effectively socialize with my peers in social setting. Teresa, Tara, Marie, and Tonya were all told that I would be sent away never to see them again almost weekly; because they did not understand that he was attempting to control them with fear of losing their only brother or the only brother that they knew.

Little did they know that the four of us had older siblings that had been adopted by our grandparents to relieve my mother of the pressures of raising a family of six alone. At that point, in our lives poverty was not the word for what our family had to deal with because we were well below the poverty level in America. The homes that we inhabited were so horrible that we had to put boards up next to ours beds to keep hundreds of rats from getting on ours beds at night. Mom provided for us as best she could, but the harsh reality was that making it would not be easy with one income. Welfare was the norm in our neighborhood. Living off the government, eating government cheese, milk, and getting IOU tickets from the neighborhood store who did not want to give us change for food stamps.

As a child, you generally know right from wrong, but a poor kid, given the opportunity to make itself happy may lean toward the wrong. At the age of five, my mom left her purse on her dresser and went to a friend's house. Her purse had over $200 worth of food stamps in it, so my sisters and I decided to have a party without her consent. Of course, me being the oldest was the ringleader I admit it. I took the fake money from the purse and we headed down the street without consent again to get whatever we wanted from the store. Well, the store manager obliged and sold us balloons, candy, games, toys, whatever we needed to have this party. We did not know that that fake money was to feed our little mouths with, not to have fun. You probably know how this ended!

Mom lost it and beat us with switches, tree limbs, ironing cords, fan belts, and fire when I tried to hide underneath the bed. Life was difficult and I was scarred from it as early as the tender age of four. Something strange happened one day, I overheard my mom on the phone with a friend telling her that it was over and that she could not take it anymore. The abuse both physical and mental had taken a toll on her body and mind, but more importantly her children were in danger and she feared that eventually he would lash out against the four of us in an attempt to hurt her even more than he had already done. At the time, I was only five so putting it all together was hard. The girls were in the one room we shared so I went to get them for breakfast assuming that mom would have it completed soon. There were garbage bags packed with clothing near the back door.

This was strange because whenever we were moving to another place, I saw the garbage bags, and mom normally told us if we had to move because we could not pay the rent or she had found something cheaper. As the girls and I walked toward the kitchen, we saw pots on the stove. My mom's husband who was my stepfather, but my sister's father was sitting in the kitchen near the window. I cannot say why, but something did not feel right about this morning, it was too quiet, no arguing, no fighting, not a sound. The next thing I heard was a blood curdling scream of I'm hot, I'm cold, I'm hot, I'm cold. My mom cooked breakfast all right; she cooked a huge pot of grits and poured them all over him to aid our escape. It happened so fast, she grabbed my youngest sister and told me to grab the garbage bags and we ran down the street as fast as we could but there was no chaser, he was still in the house with his dark complexion skin burned off to the white meat.

Getting away was nice, but we were without a home again living in the bad streets of Detroit. Eventually my mom found aid from the state, for which I am grateful. It helped keep us alive until better days would come. It was apparent in those days that survival was dependent on how far you were willing to go. Die or survive, you make the choice; we chose the latter which meant mom sacrificing herself for us. To this day, she does not know that I know, but this is an example of how deep scars go. For me the expectations became clear to me by the time I reached five.

I had become the man of the house, the disciplinarian, the one that had to do right, to get the family out of what had become a hellhole of stinky mediocrity. Philosophers of life cycles would point out that one should get responsibility based on the biological clock, but what happens to those thrust into premature adulthood before the mind is ready to assimilate the massive change from one to the other. Without the ability to gradually transition from childhood to adulthood, that individual undoubtedly will become damaged psychologically. Although they most often can overcome this broken psyche, they will never forget. Accidents do happen to children, but this is ridiculous.

My uncle cut me on the right thigh at four leaving a scar longer than my leg at the time. We found out later in life that he had gone insane from the mumps going down on him or so we were told. My sister Latonya's' thumb was caught in a washing machine ringer, you know the old type and had to have her thumb graphed to replace the skin on it. Good news though, we never had to deal with my sisters father again. A few years later after he had moved on, he caught his girlfriend and her boyfriend together, shot them both and burned the house down that he caught them in. He spent many years in jail paying the price for that one.

The bad news, a year after the escape a dog chased me over a wooden fence. To this date, I am unsure of what happened, but I do know that I woke up in the hospital after surgery to remove a splinter from my penis. These incidents only play a small part in what occurred throughout my existence that almost disabled me as a man. There is a reason a circle never ends, it is infinite as is the infinite symbol, which means that what has happened and will happen repeatedly. Maybe in different paradoxes, but nonetheless will occur to another person at some point in their lifetime. Do you believe that a child will grow into their name? Alternatively, that the name given to a child at birth will dictate their status in society, or give them strength?

Studies have shown that names play a vital role in how children are perceived, but remember, perception is not reality no matter what you have heard, if it were we all would be guilty until proven innocent. People perceive what they want to be true and attempt to substantiate it.

As dramatic as the first part of my life was what followed cut so deep that a weaker person would have checked out and committed suicide to escape from a situation that seemed hopeless. There was no light at the end of the tunnel. There was no ship coming in for us! Our life was, what it was, in that being born poor, parent uneducated, family very disjointed and unable to come together, crime, abuse, and murder, all of this before the age of five.

Outline your earliest memories

1. _____
2. _____
3. _____
4. _____
5. _____
6. _____
7. _____
8. _____
9. _____
10. _____

Scar II

Lost Childhood

The next few years bought on a myriad of new challenges. Elementary school began uneventfully, but because of finances, a move was made to send me to Alabama to live with my grandparents. This was a mistake! However, I was able to develop a relationship with my older sister Karla and Brother Jerry. Have you ever heard of child slave labor? Well this is what Jerry and I had to deal with instead of worrying about which girl liked us or which football team we would play for. Our grandfather John enlisted us to build a house for our aunt Mary who despised us because she did not like our mother. Keep in mind that Mary had a son of her own only one year younger than us, but he was excused from helping us build the house because he had light skin and we were of the darker persuasion.

This immediately drove a wedge between us. This did not sit well with me. I had survived so many things in Detroit, to be sent to work for someone I did not care for. Around this time, we were between eight and ten years old. John told us for helping him build Mary's two-story home he would pay us $10 per week. We had no choice but to accept it hell we were stuck doing it anyway. Jerry and I would be working out in the hot Alabama sun and could see Mary's son looking out of the window at us through the window of the neighboring house. Were we not as important as this cousin was? Were we inferior? To our grandparents we were because we were born from my mother.

Granted my aunt was successful in college, successful in life, and made a good living for her and her children, but nothing should come between sisters, and I mean nothing! Our generation learned from the generation before us that it was okay to not care what happens to your siblings, that it is okay to take from your siblings, that it is okay to look down on your siblings, and that it is okay to not love. Kids, especially kids from the country like to go outside and play. Jerry and I had a lot of talent, but were stuck on top of a roof while the rest of the neighborhood boys passed by laughing at us while we toiled in the sun. How can anyone in their right mind do this to children so young? Well that was the mindset then.

At the end of our second week building the house, John our grandfather gave us $10 for the weeks work. We ran to the house to take a shower so we could walk up the street to the neighborhood store. In those days, soda's were twenty-five cents, now and later's were ten cents, and stage planks were about fifteen cents so we could buy a lot of stuff with ten dollars.

Before we got of the house, our grandmother Madea who demanded $5 of the $10 stopped us. My brother who had lived with them his entire life gladly gave it to her, but I said no, this is my money for working on top of that hot roof all week! I was cursed out, beaten, and sent to one of the shared rooms we had. Why, why should I give up half of my money when it was so little anyway? From that, point on my grandmother had it out for me. One day I walked up stairs from taking a shower and overheard her talking to her next-door neighbor about me.

I stopped, what I heard was not Christian as she professed to be. She told her friend that I was nasty, evil, and did not have any home training. After I heard the last piece I slowly ascended from the stairs and she knew that I had heard everything by the way I looked at her. She hung up the phone and asked me what I was looking at. I said nothing. Soon after that incident, she called my mom to send for me, but finances prevented me from going back. I did have a couple of fond memories. Before the foundation for the house was put down, we held a neighborhood football game on the red clay dirt. Everybody came, including the kid across the street that eventually died from AIDS, turns out he was gay, but I talked him into playing anyway. Because of hard feeling, Mary's son had a bull's eye on his back.

One of the neighborhood kids broke his arm on an awesome tackle. I can still see him looking out of the window after that. Time went on, we completed the house, but it makes you wonder who your enemies and friends really are. For us the family was both friend and foe. Finally, mom had enough money to send for me so I left Alabama with a smile. After I arrived, it appeared that things had changed, but they had not. At least I could go outside and play with the neighbors since mom had a good relationship with them.

Most of the children were around my age so I dove in. I had been exposed to sex earlier in my life, but had never done anything. Who knew that an eleven-year-old girl who even at that age was a sex fiend would rape me? She invited me over to her home to play, took me in the closet even though her parents were down stairs, and told me to take my pants off. I was only eight and she was eleven. Isn't sex supposed to be for adults? I did what she said which took me down a road that has seldom been traveled, but it has been traveled. If the roles had been reversed society would have vilified me for doing that to an eight year old, but since the girl was older, the whole thing was erased as if nothing ever happened to me, yet another scar, another obstacle to overcome.

List events from age 8-12

1. _____
2. _____
3. _____
4. _____
5. _____
6. _____
7. _____
8. _____
9. _____
10. _____

Scar III

Social discomfort

Awkwardness followed like a shadow as I entered the next stage in my life. Because I was unable to develop an outgoing personality I had few friends and the ones that I did have told me that I would be there friend including a young woman that told me "If anybody ask you tell them you are my boyfriend" of course I said okay to ensure no one was offended.

How do you open up? How do you interact with young women that want to talk to you, but you have no game at all? Let them do the talking! This methodology did not always work. At one point, a girl called me a retard because she wanted me and I wanted her but all I could do is stare and hope that she would make the first move because I sure wasn't going to. I sought help and found it from my Spanish teacher Mrs. Granville. She gave me confidence to talk without being afraid, but there was still the issue of all my clothes coming from the Goodwill.

Because I had to wear my clothes repeatedly, my subconscious mind always thought someone was looking at me. To this day, I still remember the burnt orange pants and brown shirt I had to wear every week or the polyester pants that no kid wore anymore. Even in schools today, the best-dressed person, or girl remain the most popular. Teachers mean well however a large portion of them tends to misread students potential. For instance, our class took an IQ examination that I just so happen did not do to well on . I am sure she did not mean for me to hear her, but I caught her saying that I was not very bright.

Turns out, I needed glasses from day one, but money prevented my mother from getting me a pair so I wound up waiting until I joined the Army. It was not until five years after that that I got my first pair of glasses which opened my world up to so many things. Again, I shrugged off statements of non-believers, continued to wear my Goodwill clothes, and made an A in that class. Mom asked me how I managed an A in Spanish. I began sitting at the front of all my classes so I could see the board. Once the academic confidence grew, respect began grow from peers.

I began to open up some to those in my circle. Sports were a wonderful way to let loose. All that rage, stress, anger, and everything I wanted to express was let out on the football field. Everybody wanted the kid from Alabama. I soon found out that to impress or become popular, dominate in sports, America loves its athletes. There are four types of personalities: Eagle, Dove, Peacock, and Owl. The Eagle is more of a leader, conformer. The Dove is more of a follower.

The Peacock is the outgoing personality, and the owl and to know specifics and analyzes everything. Based on this I am sure you know which personality I am. The Eagle had developed from a young age and stayed with me throughout. The only things that may change or soften an eagle are life events, higher-level schooling, or training. All of us know that girls develop or mature faster than boys mature so the next scenario really was not nice for a girl to do. She asked me had I gotten my period yet and me wanting to be on top of everything and not seem like I do not know what it was so I said yes I have my period.

Everybody broke out and laughed so loud I did not know what was going on. When she stopped crying, she told me that periods were for girls and boys do not have them. Wow, I felt so stupid, but now that I look back on that episode, life is about learning, I learned to not speak unless I am sure. Something had changed; I was becoming a young man. Personality was still important, but looks became number one, then personality. Before I was able to take advantage of the new things going on in my life, the summer came and off I went back to Alabama.

Yes, I know that I need to see my older brother and sister, but to do that I still had to deal with the grandparents, the grandparents that really did not like me. I survived another boring summer, listening to the GAP band and Barry Manilow, building tree houses, and making cherry bombs with water hoses. You have to remember we had no video games or cable television in those days. There were only the three major channels and radio to provide entertainment so you had to create your own, which is not that bad considering that lack of that today.

Highlight Events age 13-15

1. _____
2. _____
3. _____
4. _____
5. _____
6. _____
7. _____
8. _____
9. _____
10. _____

Scar IV

The Transition

The girls of the family began to get crazy around the age of fifteen. All three of them left with their illiterate boyfriends for the weekend without notice. No one knew where they were, however we had our superstitions because of a large letter note left on the refrigerator. You see neither of them graduated from high school so it was hard to make out the note. My mother was very upset and it was up to me to rein them in upon their return, and did I harness them in! On Sunday morning, I saw all three of them running across the street after being dropped off by the boys they had spent the weekend. Immediately I ran to the room to get the belt to meet them.

As they came through the door, I went off on the first one telling her not to do this to mom and it is not right. She fought back while the others tried to escape by running by on the right. This is the day that I became a man, but it is also the day I lost the sibling emotion from my sisters, leaving all of us with malice for one another for years to come. Things had to change so it was decided that we would move out to California so that mom could be around the sisters she had a strong relationship with. We had gone up and down interstate 10 many times, but this trip was the most boring three days ever. Nothing but wasteland, motel 6's, more dessert, and the state of Texas, which seemed like it would never end. To this day, I do not know who told this girl that I was coming to California.

She was waiting at the apartment when I arrived. After that long trip, all I wanted to do was to shower, get something to eat, and sleep for a day or two, so I asked everyone to leave. They left, but this one girl, Amy would not leave. Her response was, I waited for you all this time, and I am not leaving. In my mind I am thinking, I don't even know you! consequently, she stayed and I slept, but when I awoke, she was still there and I knew just by looking outside that I was no longer in Alabama. It was the summer, kids were being recruited and on 84th and Main, you had a choice, you could become a CRIP or you could become a Blood. Being a country boy out in the big city of Los Angeles, I could have easily chosen to be a part of one of those gangs, but I chose neither. My choice bought the fury of 30 gang members that showed up at my apartment with guns, shotguns, and chains to find out why I told them no. Needless to say, I did not open the door because if I had all hell would have broken out and I would have probably been beaten to death.

These were the same people that one week earlier murdered the storeowner, his wife, and mother in-law in cold blood next to our apartment. I had to get a job to help buy my sisters and buy clothes for the upcoming school year. I walked down Main Street asking each store about employment. One store was willing to give me a shot. A liquor store name Ace paid minimum wage, which at that time was $4 per hour, but it did two things. It kept me off the streets and it provided much needed money for the family with me still being the only male in the home. Things were going great until the first of two robberies took place. I was working the cash register when three gunmen ran into the store shooting and yelling telling us it was a hold up.

Hell, we already knew that! It is still so clear in my mind what happened that day. The robber ran directly towards me and placed the nickel plated 45 up to my right temple and told me to empty out the cash register. At that, point calm came over me. There was no crying for my life. The only thing I said was that I never looked at you and you can take all the money, please don't shoot me because I did not see you. Whatever it was neither of us was shot that night, but we almost were shot by the LAPD who arrived well after the robbers departed the scene. The owner of the liquor store Darren called the police; they showed up, came to the door, and instructed us to come out of the store with our hands up. Wait a minute I was just robbed and I have to come out of the store with my hands up! When you deal with the LAPD, you just do it. Anyway, we both came out of the building while five police cars surrounded us as if we did it. I had an orange in my right hand that I forgot about. One of the officers told me to slowly bring my hands to the front so he could see them. I told him that it was just an orange. He repeated himself; bring your hands slowly to the front so I can see them.

I must have moved to fast because I heard a click like a gun being charged, when my boss screamed out, don't shoot he has an orange. It turned out well or I would not be writing this today, but this is a scar that I have never been able to shake. It did not take long for the second robbery to take place. Exactly one week later I was in the back room stocking liquor, I finished, and began walking up to the front to prepare for closing. Two gunmen ran into the store before I got to the front so I turned and ran to the stock room. Previously, Darren had told me to always cut the light off when I finished but I never did, but that night for some reason, I did.

The gunmen chased me to the dark room, screaming and yelling the entire time. There was no place to hide! So I crouched down behind a box that left my head in plain view, but it was so dark that he dare not take a chance because he did not know if I was armed. The robber did not know that I was looking him right in the face. My thoughts went to Darren when my assailant left. My main concern was that I did not hear anything, which normally means that someone is dead or near dead like the Asian family that had been killed next to our apartment building. Turns out, he was okay just a little shaken up. Stunned and scared I went home and found Amy, about two years later we had a son together.

I had to find a job after the debacle at the liquor store, preferably something safe with minimal chance of being robbed. My mother's boyfriend was an expert at laying carpet for the stars in Los Angeles so it seemed to be a great gig for the summer for me. Laying carpet turned out to be a very physical demanding job that wreaked havoc on the muscles. Doing that job for a long period drove Gene to drink heavily slowly drinking himself to death at the age of 40, but before he passed away, we completed a job in Beverly Hills for a major star. We were on cloud nine after that gig! On the way home, we talked and laughed about the experience.

We dropped Terry the other carpet layer off before we headed home. He offered us a drink before we left so we went in. What happened next threw us all for a loop. We heard a woman moaning and screaming for someone to fuck her. We all ran to the bedroom and found Terry's girlfriend in the buck with a guy pounding her unmercifully. Terry freaked out; they both jumped up and began running around as if the house was on fire. Terry ran out of the house in disbelief. Gene asked him if he wanted us to help him beat their asses, I was hoping that he said yes because I had never seen anything like that ever!

Shockingly, Terry kept his cool better than we did because he said no I would just leave her. In my mind, I wanted to help kill the two of them for messing around on him while he was at work. This could happen to anyone or me and it has before and will again. Gene died one month later from liver damage. It appears that drinking a pint of Black Velvet daily is not healthy. After all that, it was time to start high school. Like most young men, my goal was to play football, be popular, and have some girlfriends. That did not make Amy very happy. High school is supposed to be the time in your life, but it was not. Early on, the potential I possessed was not realized.

One of my teachers bought that to my attention. I immediately thought about the glasses because I could not see very well. It was not cool to sit in front of the class. The grades were just okay, enough to keep me out of summer school, but for college! To make a change before this was relayed to my mother I sought the assistance of the guidance counselor, she broke down each detail of my academic career from the ninth grade through the twelfth. This methodical look into why I was performing the way I was performing saved me. On that same day however, one of my classmates was shot during a drive by of Bloods in our neighborhood.

The school guards did what they could to save the remaining kids, but it was too late for Terrence as he lay outside the front door of the school soaked in blood. We signed up for this lifestyle living in California. After a while, you become desensitized to all happening around you. If I ever got the chance, I would leave California and never come back.

Relationships are fragile in High School. One minute happy, next minute broke up, that's how young relationships are. Testosterone ran through me like electricity. I needed to release the fantasies locked inside my mind. The relationship with Amy was great, but I guess like most young men good things are taken for granted. My search was for a freak, whether it be one of my sisters friends staying over or one at school. I found one such person. If my mom knew, she would call me a nasty little boy. I understand now that in the teenage years responsible coherent thinking is not one of mans forte. Hell we don't even think right at 45! I was clearly thinking with the other head. Her name was Wanda, she was a thick young sister who had a fetish for doing it time after time, and over, then saying I am pregnant when we finished.

Her mom worked as a nurse from 11-7 a.m. so I knew about 10 pm she would begin calling. She would call me minimum four times per night to come back over. She was so bad that she would call me her boyfriend's name: Oh Benny, Benny, Benny. I got busted; Amy found out about, Wanda and went the hell off. I can't blame her; I did it, but for some reason I was mad that she found out and tried to flip the script, uh, didn't work. We remained together, tried to work it out like most kids did. By doing this however, it enabled me and made me more arrogant as if I could get away with anything.

My boss Darren decided to break down the male and female sexual dynamic to me since I shared with him some of my issues. Darren had a son my age and I never met my dad so when there was a chance to get some positive influence it was welcome. His son Derrick was like most kids born with no worries, conceited, took things for granted, and wanted everything.

Darren shared the story of him buying Derrick a Corvette against his better judgment. His wife Linda who spared no expense for her children overruled him. Maybe it was too much too fast. Two months after Derrick got his car, he was given a speeding ticket for going 70 in a 55. Fifty-five was the speed limit in those days. His parents took the car for 2 weeks, but should have taken it for longer than that. He died one month later while speed racing on the shores of California. Without him, the store got busy so he hired another kid just to finish another day. Two days later, he spoke with me about sex, women, and about some of his exploits. He thought that foreplay was most important and that everything else falls into place.

Now his issue was that he was soft going in and hard coming out. I never understood that perspective with the male anatomy, but he said that it worked for him. I am not so sure it worked for his wife. About once every two weeks, my mom would pay for me to get a trim or haircut. My barber was cool as hell. His name was Bible. I never asked him why his name was Bible; I just took it for what it was. Barbers have a knack for sharing juicy stuff and why not, women do the same thing in salons. One Friday, he began talking about my bosses' wife. She was a quiet, focused businessperson, but I guess she was obviously not satisfied sexually with Darren.

From what Bible told me she would leave work, come down to the Barbershop and he would make love to her until the early morning. Do you know how hard it is to be a kid, to respect your boss, and to know his wife was sleeping with my Barber? I needed the job, so the secret was kept, never to be spoken by me. If and when he finds out it will be because she made a fatal mistake, not because she was brought down by a kid.

Scars in High School

1. _____
2. _____
3. _____
4. _____
5. _____
6. _____
7. _____
8. _____
9. _____
10. _____

Scar V

Poignant Moments

What do you do when bullets come through your kitchen window or if someone busts down your front door after being shot? Luckily, only a glass was broken in the kitchen so mom cooked dinner and we ate. The guy that was shot, well he was gunned down by Bloods; our apartment was the first one he saw so he broke it down. We had recently gotten all white furniture and a new table. That beautiful white carpet, It was all ruined with his blood going everywhere.

The table was destroyed when he collapsed and died in our living room. This was the status quo in our neighborhood. To pay the attackers back a guy from our neighborhood went to their hood, shot someone, but it only escalated with my best friend being shot in the stomach two days later while we sat on the steps in front of the apartment. We never sat on the steps again for fear of more drive-by shootings. Eventually I made the varsity football team. Times were great! I started at running back, played with four future NFL players and life was good until I broke my left hand in practice. Initially it was thought that it was sprained, but as time passed on that day, my hand began to get stiff. Later that night the pain became too much. Mom came to the rescue again and took me to the emergency room. My name was called.

At the same time, a woman stumbled through the door screaming that she had been raped. Her face was pummeled so bad that she could be hardly recognized. My hand was killing me but I told them to please take care of that woman. I felt so bad for her that my hand stopped hurting. What would trigger this type of behavior? Why would man defile woman, the most beautiful, soft, nurturing creatures on the planet? As she ran through the emergency room blooded, the scene became surreal. My heart went out to her, but my mind thought about her family. This senseless act no doubt affected her husband, children, sisters, and brothers. If I was scarred by this, I wonder what happened to her. Who knew that college was in my future? Neither my guidance counselor nor my friends could see the untapped potential inside me. When my name was called out on the loud speaker as being accepted to Alabama State University everyone just turned and looked at me. The teacher broke the silence saying congratulations.

What more could a freshman ask for? Going to school with your older sister a senior and brother a sophomore and living in the same dorm room with him. We all knew that college was stressful, but we were not told that we would have to fight to get into the dining facility every day to get breakfast, lunch and dinner. In my financial state, there was no choice but to do it. As time passed, the hunger didn't bother me anymore. I would go days without eating and lost thirty-one pounds before Thanksgiving holiday. School, partying, and fun, that's what the first year was all about until our first college dance. I had never taken a drink in my life so to get us ready for the dance my brother and his friends purchased some rotgut wine called Thunderbird and Wild Irish Rose.

We drank and drank that night. At the party, I became so inebriated that I began crawling on the floor trying to get to the door so I could throw up. Darren my brother grabbed me, and dragged me out of there and straight to the room to sleep it off. Luckily, he put me in the bottom bunk because I threw up all over the place. Meanwhile this same night on the other side of the United States in California my aunt Sue was being murdered. My oldest sister ran to my dorm room the next day crying! I was confused from the party and was hung over, but when she told me that my favorite aunt Sue had been murdered in her car after she left the club, I sobered up immediately. Turns out, she left her car doors open; someone waited in the back seat and strangled her with her panty hose.

To this date, no one has found this person. We can only hope that justice got him for something else! To quote Samuel L. Jackson in all of his movies "Enough is Enough" I dropped out of college, returned to California where I met my future wife and joined the Army. We met in High School but she was one year behind me. You know what they say marry young, divorce young and that's exactly what happened. I met Patrice by way of my sister. To this day, the series of events that followed have never left me. Patrice and I were only 19 and 18 when we were married. Most young men have no idea what plans they have, but I made a critical decision early. At nineteen, I enlisted into the United States Army.

Soon after enlistment, I had orders for Nuremburg, Germany. Patrice was still in High School so we would have to wait until she graduated before she could join me in overseas. It was a long nine months before I would see her. On many occasions, I attempted to make contact but the six-hour difference was difficult. Every time I called, she was out with her friends, her mom and sister told me, but I thought different. I was fortunate to catch her at home one time and we talked about getting an annulment if she had been seeing someone. She declined and said that everything was okay, that she did not have anything to hide.

I implored her to not come; please do not come over here if you have been unfaithful because I had been very faithful the entire time. She came anyway. It had been so long that we made love four times a day. On the third day, something started coming out of my penis. It was a white liquid and it hurt while I was urinating. I thought maybe it was the stress from having sex, so much so I waited another four days. By then it was unbearable. In the Army there was a place called sick call, so I went one morning. The Physician on call said I had it, I'm like, have what? You have gonorrhea! Not only was I shocked, but my boss was on sick call as well. Obviously, he was not a good supervisor because it spread around the barracks like wildfire. It appeared that what I feared was true.

My supervisor excused me for the day so that I could have time to speak with my wife. On the way, home thoughts keep going through my mind. How would I react? How is she going to take it? Moreover, would my marriage be truncated by an affair that I foresaw before she even arrived? As I walked through the door, she ran to the bathroom and kneeled over the toilet crying. She knew that I knew.

Calm came over me. Maybe it was because of all I had gone through that has prepared me for this moment. I told her that I had gonorrhea and she broke down. We did not talk for three days. She cooked dinner that Friday, but all I could think of was if she was trying to poison me? No, she was trying to make things better. The food really looked good and I was hungry, but she had betrayed my trust and now wants to get back in with me! I don't think so. She got upset that the food was not eaten so she took the plate and hit me in the back of the head with it, breaking the plate. She was not satisfied that it broke she wanted to damage me forever so with the sharp end of the broken plate she hit an artery in the back of my head giving me a thirty stitch gash. All of my clothes were destroyed with the amount of blood coming out of me. My shirt, pant, and tennis shoes were ruined, but what was worse, my life was about to expire from the lack of blood flowing through my body. She panicked, and I ran to the cabstand to try to get to the hospital as quick as possible. Every cabby refused because of the amount of blood.

In their eyes, their cab was more important than my life. I struggled back to the apartment and as I entered the door, a Military Policeman offered to take me to the hospital. I ruined his jeep, but he did his job to serve and protect. If he had been selfish, I would not be here today. The doctor gave me Thirty-two stitches with nothing to sedate me. After surgery, the police met me in my room to ask questions about what led to the incident. I went to live in the barracks for fear of her freaking out again. Law officials asked me whether I wanted to press charges, but being young and stupid, I declined. When we got back together, she told me that she was pregnant. Me being the kind of man that wanted to make it work, I stayed with her for another year and a half. Why, I just wanted to know why. Her excuse was that she went out, got high, had too much drugs and four guys had their way with her. I know what you are thinking, who is the father of the baby?

It is so strange how everyone knows what is going on in your marriage but you. The girl slept with two of my closest associates. You know it's bad when you come home and there is a man sitting in your bedroom, the kid in the crib and the wife sitting on the bed. Imagine the kind of thoughts going through my mind. During the first break up after the gonorrhea incident, she moved in with a friend of hers who happened to be married to another guy in my company. Bad move on her part. She slept with her husband and had his baby, but tried to pen it on me. We did not have the Maury show back in those days. Football was a way for me to relieve some tension so it was great to be able to use that outlet to facilitate the healing process. Unfortunately, the word had gone all around Nuremburg, Germany that my wife was a freak. Whispers began as soon as I hit the field, but the intensive focus on the football field shielded me from the callous remarks from the crowd. No matter, I would be rid of her at the first opportunity, which came two months later.

After the baby was born she went back home to California to live with her mother. Up to this point, Life had taught me one thing, Never, ever trust a woman. After all, I had gone through Jeff; a good friend of mine met the woman of his life during my first assignment in Nuremberg, Germany. The German woman, Black American male dynamic was something to see. It seemed as though they really got into each other, but most of all there was no color barrier in Germany. Now a seasoned vet will tell you that all the German girls want is to get back to America and divorce you.

The true believers in love will tell you that this theory is flawed and cynical. I have my own theory that encompasses a little bit of both. Jeff was madly in love with Tessa. He introduced her to all of us as his lady. In those days courtships developed quickly with one thought, marriage. Jeff soon proposed to Tessa, we all knew this was coming! He ran to his car every day after we got off work to get to her, and her to him. The date was set for July 15th so we all prepared for the big day. For the bachelor party we rented sex videos and bought a couple of strippers for him.

The party was hot! The strippers showed up, we popped in one of the videos and kicked it off. Five minutes into the video, the party stopped with a thud. Jeff saw his fiancé on the video sucking a man's penis and went to pieces. The marriage was over, but who would explain this to Tessa? That would be me. Number one, hiding things going into a marriage is not good, but this was total deception. She wasn't who he thought she was. Jeff lost thirty pounds after that night and never regained the swagger he had before this happened.

Don't ask me why, but I invited Patrice to move to Fort Benning, Georgia, in attempt to make it work one more time. Trying almost cost me my life. This was the weakest point in my life. Life sucked and I did not know whom to confide in at this tender age. In an attempt to reach out, I slit my wrist, as it was the only way for me to express myself. I was still non-talkative and unable to unearth the skill of interaction to defeat my demons. I was taught to let it out the one week I spent in the hospitals mental ward. Shortly after this episode, she arrived to Georgia. As we were trying to work through it periodically, she would go out by herself and I would go out by myself because we did not have a baby sitter. One Friday night I went out, but came back at 11:55, because I was dog-tired.

You ever have that feeling that someone was standing over you in your sleep? Whatever it was it saved my life. She was so upset that she went into the kitchen, grabbed the largest butcher knife I'd ever seen, ran towards me, and began stabbing me. By the grace of god, my eyes opened as the first blow came down. My natural reaction was to put my hands up to stop the knife. My hands suffered six one-inch deep stab wounds before I was able to subdue her and take the knife away. Before I knew it, I snapped! I had never hit a woman before, but the survival instincts kicked in when my brain felt life was about to be taken.

I went the hell off, Throwing punches as if she was a man, screaming and hollering like I had gone insane. It was over; it was time for her to go back to California. This woman was so vindictive that she tried to pour sugar into my gas tank, but she was so stupid that she poured it inside the cap not the actual hole that the gas goes in. That's what she gets for not putting gas in the car.

Damn if that same supervisor somehow received the same assignment as I and wound up in charge of me again. This was terrible! He was a bad leader, could not keep his mouth shut, and did not lead by example. His uniform was never ironed; his boots resembled a chocolate bar before you ate it. One day we had an inspection. I was second in charge so my supervisor was inspected first, then me. The First Sergeant asked my supervisor who was in charge because your subordinates look better than you. The entire company was stunned by the comment, but he took it especially hard. His tenure with us ended shortly afterwards.

He was dismissed for lack of leadership and I was put in charge of the seven-man team to whip it into shape. No one would want to jump right into another marriage after what I had gone through, but life does not care what you want. As the designated leader and responsible adult, I volunteered to pick up some of my peers who did not have a car and lived off post.

This went on for months upon months that I drove five miles back and forth to help them out. Eventually we would all start hanging out together, having barbeques, fight parties, football parties, and just all kinds of stuff. Funny, I was still married, but my future wife was married to one of the guys I was picking up and I did not know it. As I have said, life does not care, it just happens. Nothing happened, we did not have an affair, never even discussed any type of relationship issues. We've been talking about trigger mechanisms that affect the course of your life. This trigger led me to my wife of twenty-one years Charlotte. One thing led to another and we all began getting high on weed every day, drinking Gin, and eating skins. We soon graduated to crack, cocaine, and acid. That was our daily ritual until one of our crew was busted on drugs. After that, all of us were suspected of using. Each member of the group was tested and all came up hot, but me.

Misery followed in all of our personal lives. My wife was sent back to California, we finally divorced, the guy I was telling you about that was married to my current wife; he left over night after he was released from the service with no notice, never to be heard from again. My best friend Stanley got so high when he was busted that he thought I was with him when someone knocked him in the head with a 2x4. He woke up in jail, got one call and it was me. I told him that we were not together, that I was with Charlotte, but he did not believe me. Drugs make the mind do weird things. It took Charlotte to tell him as we visited him in jail that I never left her side that night and he only imagined that I was in the fight with him and ran. Even in those days if you did not have two incomes, your lifestyle would have to change when those events occur. Arrangements were made for me to live with one of my nearby friends and she moved in with one of hers. Since I required very little, whatever I could do to help anyone I did. That's just who I was at the time. If you needed money and I had it fine. Need a car for the day, great here you go! Charlotte came to me one day because she had no transportation for work. Of course, I said yes, but please bring it back as soon as you get off from work. We both had it rough, which made us both see one another differently.

Maybe me being a gentlemen actually appealed to her, but was I ready for this? We hooked up and a year and a half later, we decided to get married, a big step after the debacle in Germany. Before the wedding date, I skipped out of town, and drove to California like a coward, afraid of dedicating my life to another woman after being screwed over. The long drive gave me the opportunity to analyze and assess whether this would be good for me. About the time, I arrived in California my mind had changed 15 times, but I came to my senses.

The overwhelming factor was whether she was a good woman or not and whether she could be trusted. Never again would I be scarred like before. I drove back to Fort Benning, Georgia another three long days. When I arrived, she was sleeping on the coach waiting for me. She asked me what made me come back. The trigger was love. However, don't get it twisted! It takes more than love to make a twenty-one year marriage work. From the outside looking in many marriages look perfect and if a couple told you that it was they would be lying! A few of my readers asked me why I listed marriage as a scar. Well from the beginning, marriage is great right? You have your beautiful wedding, wonderful reception, then wake up the next day to real life. Bills for the wedding, discovering one another's little quirks that you did not know about because it was cleverly hidden during the dating phase. Once the novelty wears off most couples wonder if they made the right choice to have an elaborate wedding rather than go down to the judge and just have him do it. Marriage is a wonderful thing if it is done for the right reason. Those that jump into marriage just because he asked you or for the guy who has cold feet and does not want to back out now, it may be the beginning a scar that lasts a lifetime. As beautiful as they are, marriage often fails more than fifty percent of the time due to a myriad of reasons, but mainly due to infidelity, finances, and irreconcilable differences. They just were not who you thought they were!

Ask yourself, does she mind if you leave your socks on the floor at night? I am sure she does. Does she hate it when you pass gas? You are not truly one until both of you have past gas around one another. Yes, this sounds gross, but it is real. What about washing dishes? Have you asked her if she wants you to help with responsibilities around the house? Men, does your fiancé nag you right now? If so, do you think that it will lesson when you get married? Sorry guys it will not! Ladies does your man have many friends that he hangs out with all the time? You may need to talk about this before you jump the broom. His boys are important to him so if you are unable to compromise, and communicate this to him, you are in trouble!

Guys, is your woman controlling before you even get married? A lot of them are, but most times for good reason. The bottom line is, compromise, communication, sharing your past, and writing down your individual quirks before marriage will save you some time and heartache. Through all of this, if you and your mate have the ability to tolerate your differences your relationship will flourish rather than leave scars.

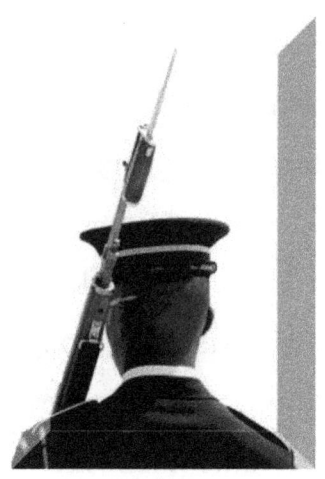

Scar VI

The Career

It was unbelievable that through all of this that I was able to keep all that drama from affecting my performance at work. My career flourished, Rewards followed, promotions, and recognition, but with all this come responsibility. It is true that soldiers do more before nine, than most people do all day. The norm is to awaken daily at 5:30 am to prepare for physical training in case the call came for combat. When you choose this profession, you have chosen to support and defend the nation against all foreign and domestic threats. What is a leader? Some people think that leaders are born, however any rational person knows that the environment, education, and events, are major factors that shape how and if a person will have the ability to lead. The first ten years of my career were wonderful Hardly any responsibility, just doing my job, with only my success in mind, but after a grueling tour at Fort Benning, Georgia I was assigned to Athens, Greece.

It's bad to live in fear of having your head blown off. During my time in Athens, Greece, I had to have a sense of heightened awareness or a bomb could be placed underneath your car. There was a group called November- 17 who had it out for Americans in Greece. To avoid situations alternate routes had to be taken daily. Uniforms were not allowed in public, and early days and nights were mandatory. All of this because at some point, these safety measures were disregarded and a bus full of service men and women was bombed leaving twenty people injured. Talk about keeping your head on a swivel.

What this incident did was prepare those of us scheduled for deployment to Fort Hood hands on training in intense situations. Four months later, it would serve us well when Desert Storm kicked off. I know war; it is a filthy, austere, awful place.

War damages family to the core. The military always speaks of causalities of war, but rarely do they discuss the family unit destroyed by it. At the end of combat operations, thousands of marriages ended as a result. Broken homes, destroyed lives, and hardship ensued as women came back pregnant, men came back to empty homes, wives who had gotten pregnant since they departed, and divorce papers. War truly is hell.

Some people get peach assignments and I admit that some of mine were cake, but when I was assigned to recruiting it changed my personality from an easy going introvert to a forceful out going extrovert only when I had to. It was sort of like acting my way to success. This was the toughest job on the planet at the time. Long hours, constantly being told no, going from hero to zero, and failing for the first time in my life. Grueling cannot describe how intense and degrading at times those assignments made me feel.

To try to explain it better look at this analogy: pretend that you are responsible for thirty-five people that respect you one day then the next day your only responsibility is yourself and recruiting the future of the armed forces. In the end the Gold recruiting badge followed, but not without tears.

It was finally time to leave so I walked outside the door and kissed the ground and thanked God that I made it without ruining my career. To try my mettle the Army sent me to Alaska the coldest place on the earth. Upon arrival, I quickly learned what everyone had told me about this assignment. Cold, Cold, Cold, six months of light, six months of dark, and one of the highest rates of suicide because of the darkness. Thirty-five below zero is not what I call a fun physical training session, but to get qualified as an arctic soldier it had to be done. One night in a tent out in the wilderness with temperature minimum 35 below zero without coming inside. Do that and you are qualified. Besides being one of the coldest places on the planet, Alaska was awesome. It was time to go again, but Before I arrived for my assignment in Texas, I had to complete training to prepare me for the assignment. While on assignment at now defunct Fort Benjamin Harrison, Indiana, my 1980 Cutlass LS broke down with a bad radiator.

It was too far to walk back to the post so I called for another Non-commissioned offer to pick me up. She arrived about an hour later. There was a little restaurant nearby so we went over to it to try to get some help. Were we in for the shock of our lives?

The first thing I noticed was that that all eyes were focused on me. I slid over to the phone booth to call the NCO in charge. While inside the booth, I overheard one of the men asking one of the other men, what I was doing in there with that nice looking white woman, and that he was going to his car to get his gun and shoot that nigger.

I completed that call quickly and got the hell out of there! Two months later, my son suffered a fate worse than I could imagine. A woman crawled through his window, and stabbed him thirty-two times in the head, neck, and shoulder area killed him at eight years old. While grieving, I awoke at 3 a.m. one morning and he was standing beside my bed. He asked me if he could go with his mom and me. I broke down, trying to be strong for him even in death and told him that he could not. I told him to go to Jesus and we will meet you there. He began crying because he could not understand what had happened to him, but he slowly turned with his head down, crying and said that he loved us. It was a dream so vivid that is scarred me for the rest of my life! However, I now have a glimpse into the scar of losing a child. He does not know that I ran to his bed and slept with him for the remainder of that night. Though it was a dream, it made me cherish my babies more.

It was time to move on to the great state of Texas, back to a recruiting battalion as a Senior Personnel Management Supervisor.

If I had known the future, I would have never gone. The stress was like a forty-pound rucksack placed on my back from the beginning. I quickly cracked under the pressure, went to the doctor who prescribed anti-anxiety medicine to help deal with everything being thrown at me. I regret accepting that prescription over counseling. In this case, some form of counseling would have been appropriate rather than attacking it with medications. The almost twenty years of soldiering had taken its toll, but I still had one more assignment to go, it would be the worst of them all. The Iraqi war was around the corner.

No one has more respect for what the armed forces does for our country, but more goes on than you know. The military is just like a large corporation. You start at the bottom and earn your way up the ladder. Great concept, but if you are injured you are vilified as someone trying to get over on the system. I was injured late in my career after leading from the front all of my life. The last assignment of my career was Fort Campbell, Kentucky on the border of Clarksville, Tennessee. All of the top ranked Non commissioned officers met with the top ranked Non- commissioned officer for the installation to conduct morning physical training and to get his philosophy on leadership. Before the run began, he separated those with what they called a physical profile and could not run.

What happened after that was very unprofessional. He walked up to me and asked me how I going to lead my people if I could not run? He then said that I was useless and a waste of my stripes. Wow! After eighteen years of service, this is what it had come to, a berating in front of all my pears. One year later, I deployed with a group of 35 soldiers to Iraq. We crossed over the border at the bottom of the IRAQ and went all the way to the top in Mosul. I was awarded the Bronze Star Medal for combat operations. I guess even though I had an injury that kept me from running, I was still able to lead! 35 soldiers went over there and 35 came back. That was my proudest moment. Shortly after, I retired into the civilian sector at the age of thirty-nine.

Like most veterans I struggled to deprogram mentally from being Hooah-Hooah, gun-ho everyday to trying to smoothly assimilate back into civilian life without being perceived as arrogant or overbearing. War had left me a gift, the inability to sleep. For the first year after I retired there was a raging battle going on inside the sub consciousness of my mind nightly. Fighting, cursing, acting out, and hitting Charlotte in my sleep and waking up to eat at 2 am every night. It has been said that being in the military is kind to being in prison because you become institutionalized due to the controlled environment and time spent in one organization. For me this rang true, but I eventually was able to relax, let everything go, and finally the dreams of war began to subside. They come back periodically. Charlotte put some holy oil on my head hoping to rid my dreams of demons. She said that the voice coming from me was not mine, but still I had overcome the worst dreams leaving me feeling somewhat ordinary again.

Career Stumbling Blocks

1. _____
2. _____
3. _____
4. _____
5. _____
6. _____
7. _____
8. _____
9. _____
10. _____

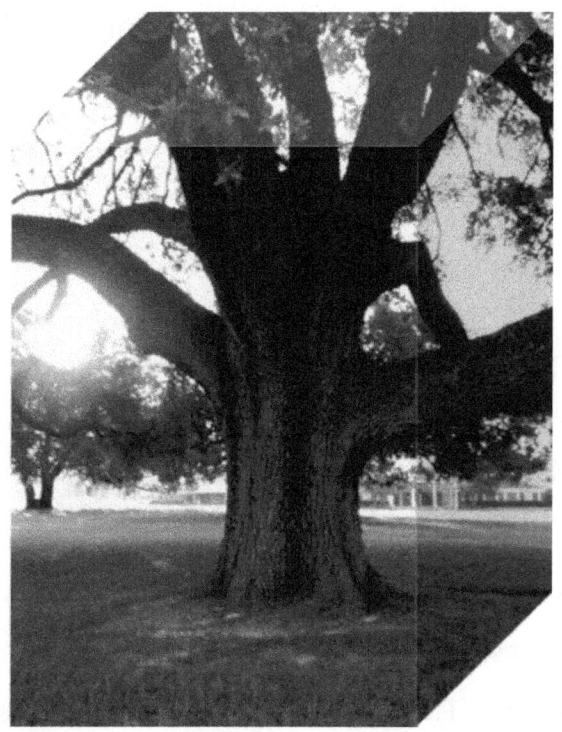

Scar VII

The Foundation

What you have read is a series of events that could have been prevented with proper intervention. Granted not all of them could have been stopped, but the trigger mechanisms had already cemented my fate for every battle to follow. At the time, I did not know that I was not fighting alone. As I look back, blessed was not the word, it was favored. Every step of the way a spiritual guide had bought me to this point through all the major setbacks, financial problems, and the inner struggle I had within myself to find a way no matter the consequence. It is my hope that you were able to see some correlation between my life and yours, those events are always triggered by something, they do not just happen.

They will happen again, and again unless you recognize that you have a choice. You have hope if you listen to yourself and those trying to mentor you. Those that have come before you have lived it, listen. It is the circle of infinity, the factor of human nature that in itself is flawed. Finally, history is an account of the past, failure to respect and learn from it is the acceptance of events reoccurring. The emotional and physical scars cannot always be avoided, but can be concealed by selective accouterment.

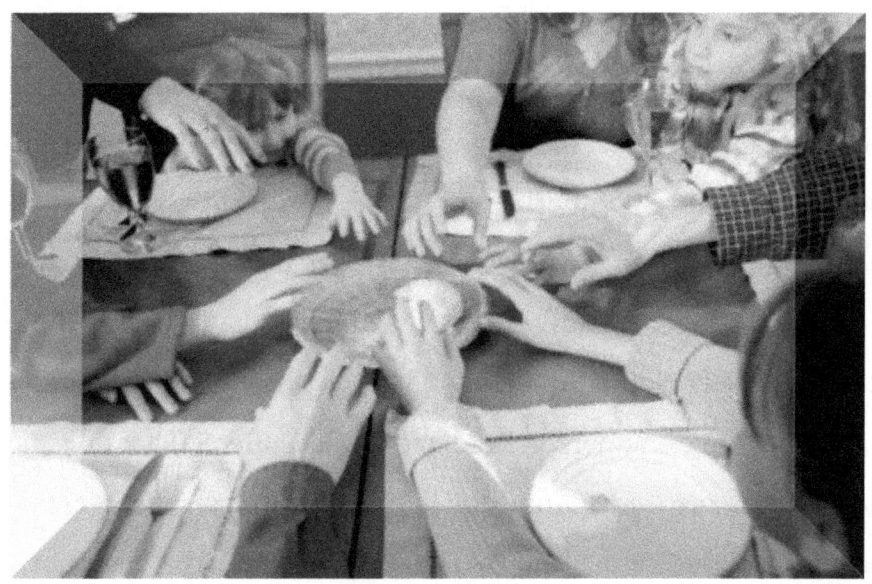

Scar VIII

The Dysfunctional Family

Get your family in order! The hurtful remarks made by the older generation will scar the younger family members forever. It has no place and it serves no purpose. As time passes with no contact, family becomes more like long lost friends. There is no emotional connection when this happens. Selfishness within the family core has no place. You may be wondering who is responsible for ensuring the family legacy survives. The responsibility falls upon the entire group, but is the responsibility of the elders to bring it all together, to strengthen the relationships.

The young are impressionable. They mimic what they see. If you curse, they curse. If you wear your pant down near your ankles, they will as well. Hit your wife or husband in front of them, they will remember! Trauma and pain from parents' and their siblings, actions, words, and attitudes can lead to the division of the family unit. Does your family really care if they see each other? Some do not. As families grow older, life has a way of sending one person here and another there. That does not mean out of site out of mind for families. Twenty-seven years have passed one career and two deaths, now family I have not heard from that want to contact me. Oh wait, someone died and left some money that's why.

Hey, that is the way some would rather it be, but why? Now that our aunts are getting up in age, I know they wonder if we are coming to their funeral should we outlive them. There is a good chance that most of us will not. After our funerals, everyone should say see you next time someone passes away, but no one does. Existing like this is sad, but true. There are no emotional ties to them. They made it a point to torment us during our early years. It got to the point that they wanted to visit my family in a couple of states, but since the trust level was not, I pretended that

I was not home.

This family is emotionally empty and not one of them has stepped up to discuss anything about the past so that we all could go beyond the issues that have gone unanswered. Why does family become jealous or preoccupied with the status of another family member? Every success story is a feather for the family; it should not be a wedge between them. Celebrate in success and rejoice, someday it may be yours. It burns my britches when a man or woman allows their spouse to make them disassociate themselves from his family. Normally, the male begins associating with his wife's side of the family after marriage more than his own, and then the male has to salvage some of his senses and start communicating with his family. This goes both ways, but more often than not, the male is drawn away from his family.

Do you live around the corner from your sibling or family and have not seen them in a year? I have, do not know why, it is in walking distance with no contact. Does your family rather text you than talk to you? Mine does. This is just my perspective, but there are deep seeded untold stories that have been hidden for generations. This is a classic case of a family unable to develop intimate relationships with one another, which carried over to the next generation who carry on this sorrowful way. I missed my grandfather funeral and did not feel a thing. I missed my aunt's funeral and did not feel a thing. You ask why? It's easy when the older generation does not make a point to get to know their nephews and nieces.

Vicious aunts and unfocused, non supporting uncles that abused us mentally telling us we would never grow up to be anything, or you are fat, or would be in prison by 18. Then as we grew older those very words turned on them when their kids became what they envisioned for us. Besides, my grandfather pulled a shotgun on me when I was only twelve years old because he thought that I had stolen money from his chest that he kept in his room with thousands of one-dollar coins hidden in it. He was old school so the bank did not make much since to him, that was his rational for keeping it there, but he soon discovered after I ran away that he had misplaced one of his bags of money. My brother found me and explained what took place, but I was afraid to go back into that home. Why did he think that I had stolen from him? There were three other kids in the home at the time and two of them were older than me. Later that day I found enough courage to go back, home. My grandfather apologized, but that could not remove the image of a 12-gauge shotgun being pointed in my face by my grandfather nonetheless. In a normal family, brothers and sisters look after one another, but in my mother's generation, sisters charge their sisters for rent, steal from each other, and look out for themselves. I had had enough when my aunt went through my wife's purse while we were on vacation. Who will be the matriarch? Who will be the one family member, either man or woman to grab hold and bring the family unit together no matter what the geographical issues are? Maybe the lack of a matriarch is the main cause of torn families. Maybe the lack of strength at what should be the foundation has led to the numerous families crumbling beneath itself. I was reminded of this when a friend of mine lost the matriarch of their family.

Not only did that family find comfort within itself, but also the love overflowed from visitors, friends, and onlookers that succumbed to the generational love flowing throughout the entire building. This family did not just gather when someone passed away in the family, they came together to fellowship with one another regularly to ensure the family unit had that third bond (God) wrapped around its unit. Admittedly, I have always been cynical of almost anything, but I found proof that there are families out there that share what cannot be broken through hardship, finances, or death. Finally, kids are very keen, never play favorites, give them purpose, and treat them all the same because one of them may grow up to write a book. Let us look at how to overcome the effects of a dysfunctional family and how to make your family thrive emotionally.

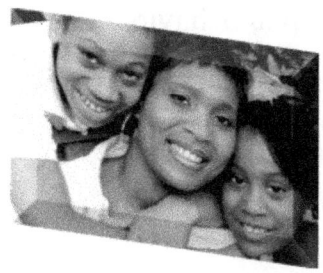

HOW CAN YOU OVERCOME THE EFFECTS OF A DYSFUNCTIONAL FAMILY?

Regardless of the source of dysfunction, you have survived. You have likely developed a number of valuable skills to get you through tough circumstances.

Consequently, it is important to first stop and take stock. You may find that much of what you learned in your family is valuable.

Many of the survival behaviors you developed are your best assets. For example, people who grow up in dysfunctional families often have finely tuned empathy for others; they are often very achievement-oriented and highly successful in some areas of their lives; they are often resilient to stress and adaptive to change. In examining changes, you may want to make in yourself, it is important not to lose sight of your good qualities.

Patience is necessary! Negative effects from growing up in dysfunctional families often stem from survival behaviors that were very helpful when you were growing up, but may become problematic in your adult life. Remember that you spent years learning and practicing your old survival skills, so it may take awhile to learn and practice new behaviors.

Get Help. In most dysfunctional families children tend to learn to doubt their own intuition and emotional reactions. Often outside support provides an objective perspective and much-needed affirmation, which will help you learn to trust your own reactions. Help or support can take many forms: individual counseling, therapy groups such as Survivors of Incest or Adult Children of Dysfunctional Families (ACODF), and self-help groups such as Adult Children of Alcoholics (ACOA), Alanon, or Codependents Anonymous (CODA). Kansas State Counseling Services offers a variety of therapy groups each semester.

Learn to Identify and Express Emotions. Growing up in a dysfunctional family often results in an exaggerated attention to others' feelings and a denial of your own feelings and experiences. While this often results in very good sensitivity to others, you may have neglected sensitivity to yourself. Stop each day and identify emotions you are or have been experiencing. What triggered them? How might you affirm or respond to them? Try keeping a daily feelings journal.

Be selective in sharing your feelings with others. You may not find it helpful to share all of your feelings. In sharing your feelings with others take small risks first, and then wait for a reaction. If the responses seem supportive and affirming, try taking some larger risks.

Allow Yourself to Feel Angry About What Happened.

Forgiveness is a very reasonable last step in recovery, but it is a horrible first step. Children need to believe in and trust their parents; therefore, when parents behave badly, children tend to blame themselves and feel responsible for their parents' mistakes. These faulty conclusions are carried into adulthood, often-leaving guilt, shame, and low self-esteem. When you begin with trying to forgive your parents, you will likely continue to feel very badly about yourself.

Placing the responsibility for what happened during your childhood where it belongs, i.e., with the responsible adults, allows you to feel less guilt and shame and more nurturance and acceptance toward yourself.

It is usually helpful to find productive ways to vent your anger. This can be done in support groups or with good friends. Try writing a letter to one or both of your parents and then burning the letter. You may want to talk with your parents directly about what happened.

If you decide to do this, it is important to keep your goal clear. Do you want to encourage change and work for a better relationship, or are you trying to get even or hurt them back? Pursuing revenge frequently results in more guilt and shame in the long run. Holding on to anger and resentment indefinitely is also problematic and self-defeating. Focusing on old resentments can prevent growth and change.

Begin the Work of Learning to Trust Others. Take small risks at first in letting others know you. Slowly build up to taking bigger risks. Learning who to trust and how much to trust is a lengthy process. Adult children from dysfunctional families tend to approach relationships in an all-or-nothing manner. Either they become very intimate and dependent in a relationship, or they insist on nearly complete self-sufficiency, taking few interpersonal risks. Both of these patterns tend to be self-defeating.

Frequently, children of dysfunctional families continue to seek approval and acceptance from their parents and families. If these people could not meet your needs when you were a child, they are unlikely to meet your needs now. Recognize your parents' limitations while still accepting whatever support they can offer. Seek your support from other adults. Practice saying how you feel and asking for what you need. Don't expect people to guess -- **tell** them. This step will likely require much effort.

Practice Taking Good Care of Yourself. Frequently, survivors of dysfunctional families have an exaggerated sense of responsibility. They tend to overwork and forget to take care of themselves. Try identifying the things you really enjoy doing, and then give yourself permission to do at least one of these per day. Work on balancing the things you should do with the things you want to do. Balance is a key word for people who've grown up in dysfunctional families.

Identify areas you tend to approach compulsively: Drinking? Eating? Shopping? Working? Exercising? How might you approach this in a more balanced fashion? One of the best things you can do for your mental and emotional well-being is to take good physical care of yourself. Do you eat a good healthy balanced diet? Do you get regular exercise?

Begin to Change Your Relationships with Your Family.

Keep the focus on yourself and your behavior and reactions. Remember, you cannot change others, but you can change yourself. Work on avoiding entanglements in your family Õs problems. Alanon calls this "detachment." Counseling or support is usually crucial when trying to change family relationships. You are fighting a lifetime of training in getting hooked into their problems, usually including large doses of guilt.

It is also important to be patient with your family. They may find it difficult to understand and accept the changes they see in your behavior. While most families can be workable, undoubtedly there are some rare families who are far too dangerous or abusive to risk further contact.

Read. Many books provide helpful information about dysfunctional families and strategies for recovering from their effects. Here is a short list of some we recommend:

Forward, S. (1989). Toxic parents: Overcoming their hurtful legacy and reclaiming your life. New York: Bantam Books.

Gravitz, H.L. and Bowden, J.L. (1985). Guide to recovery: A book for adult children of alcoholics. Holmes Beach, FL: Learning Publications.

Beattie, M. (1987). Codependent no more: How to stop controlling others and start caring for yourself. New York: Harper and Row.

Gil, E. (1983) Outgrowing the pain: A book for and about adults abused as children. San Francisco: Launch Press.

Bass, E. and Davis, L. (1988). The courage to heal: A guide for women survivors of child sexual abuse. New York: Harper & Row.

REFERENCES

Vannicelli, M. (1989). *Group psychotherapy with adult children of alcoholics: treatment techniques and counter transference.* New York: Guilford Press.

Forward, S. (1989). *Toxic parents: Overcoming their hurtful legacy and reclaiming your life.* New York: Bantam Books.

This help yourself originally written and developed in 1993 by Sheryl A. Benton, Ph.D., Counseling Services; updated/modified for the internet in 1997 by Dorinda J. Lambert, Ph.D..

Patriarch

Male Head of family: a man who is the head of a family or group

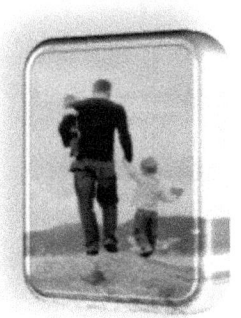

Matriarch

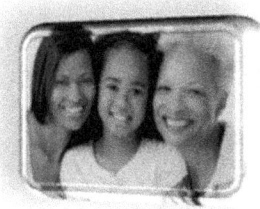

Woman head of family: a woman who is recognized as being the head of a family, community, or people

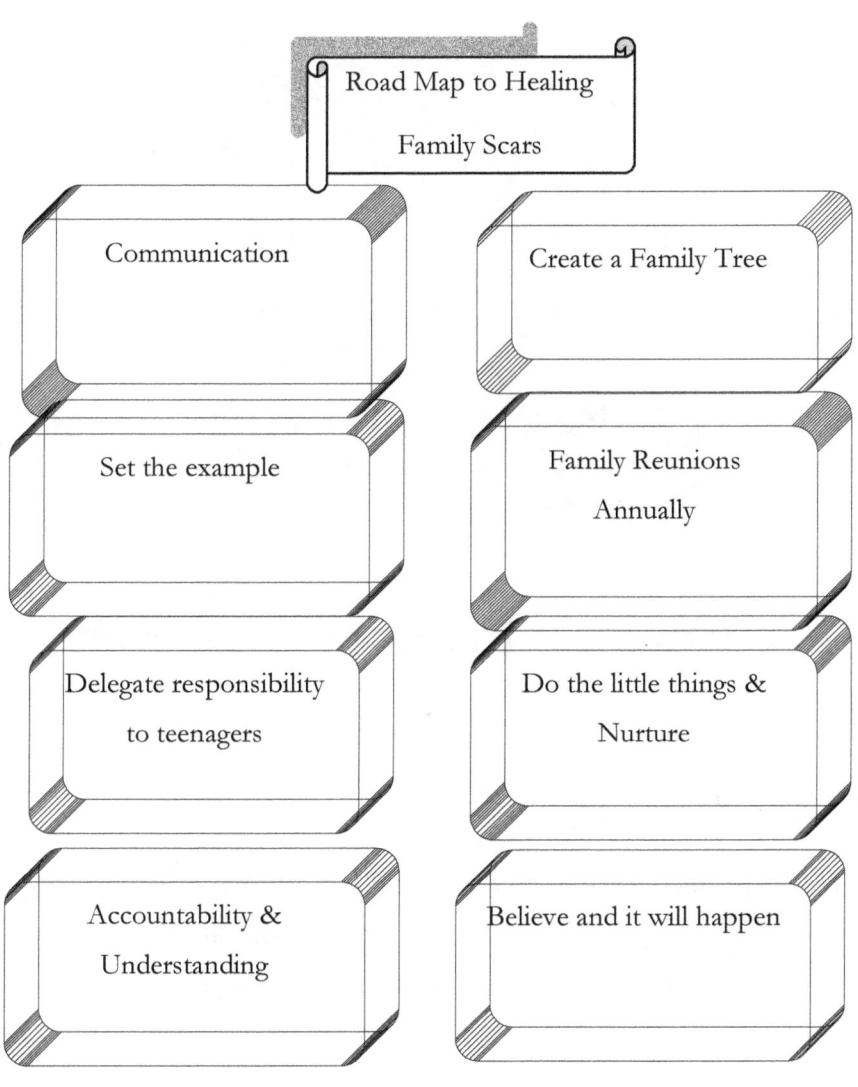

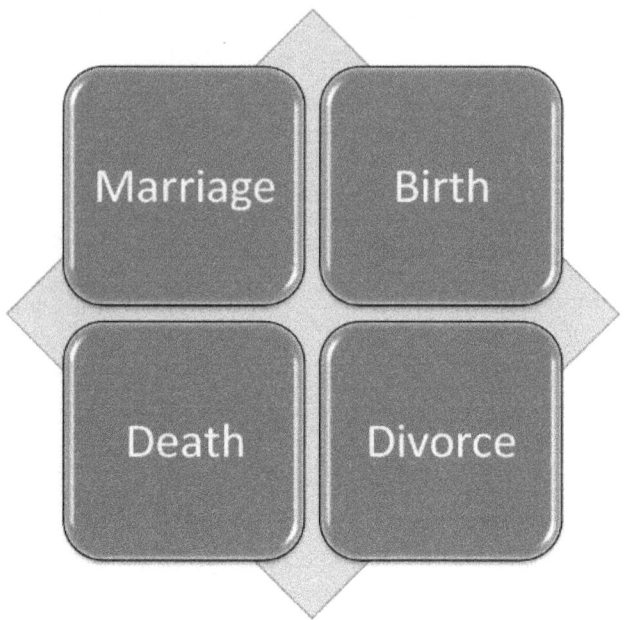

Every event is triggered by an event

IX

Philosophy of determinism

Determinism necessarily entails that humanity or individual humans may not change the course of the future and its events (a position known as fatalism); however, some determinists believe that the level to which human beings has influence over their future is itself merely dependent on present and past. Causal determinism is associated with, and relies upon, the ideas of materialism and causality. Some of the main philosophers who have dealt with this issue are Marcus Aurelius, Omar Khayyám, Thomas Hobbes, Baruch Spinoza, Gottfried Leibniz, David Hume, Baron d'Holbach (Paul Heinrich Dietrich), Pierre-Simon

Laplace, Arthur Schopenhauer, William James, Friedrich Nietzsche, Albert Einstein, Niels Bohr, and, more recently, John Searle, Ted Honderich, and Daniel Dennett.

Mecca Chiesa notes that the probabilistic or selectionistic determinism of B.F. Skinner comprised a wholly separate conception of determinism that was not mechanistic at all. A mechanistic determinism would assume that every event has an unbroken chain of prior occurrences, but a selectionistic or probabilistic model does not.

The nature of determinism

The exact meaning of the term *determinism* has historically been subject to rigorous scrutiny and several interpretations. Some people, called *Incompatibilists*, view determinism and free will as mutually exclusive. The belief that free will is an illusion is known as *Hard Determinism*. Others, labeled *Compatibilists*, (or *Soft Determinists*) believe that the two ideas can be coherently reconciled. Incompatibilists who accept free will but reject determinism are called *Philosophical Libertarians* — not to be confused with Political Libertarians. Some feel it refers to the metaphysical truth of independent agency, whereas others simply define it as the feeling of agency that humans experience when they act. Many will agree that determinism is the theory that human choices and actions can be determined from external causes; but free will is the theory that human choices and actions are determined by internal causes: that an individual is the prime mover of his life.

Ted Honderich, in his book *How Free Are You? - The Determinism Problem* gives the following summary of the theory of determinism:

In its central part, determinism *is* the theory that our choices and decisions and what gives rise to them is effects. What the theory comes to therefore depends on what effects are taken to be... [I]t is effects that seem fundamental to the subject of determinism and how it affects our lives.

Varieties of determinism

Causal (or *nomological*) determinism is the thesis that future events are necessitated by past and present events combined with the laws of nature. Such determinism is sometimes illustrated by the thought experiment of Laplace's demon. Imagine an entity that knows all facts about the past and the present, and knows all natural laws that govern the universe. Such an entity might be able to use this knowledge to foresee the future, down to the smallest detail. Simon-Pierre Laplace's determinist "dogma" (as described by Stephen Hawking) is generally referred to as "scientific determinism" and predicated on the supposition that all events have a cause and effect and the precise combination of events at a particular time engender a particular outcome. This causal determinism has a direct relationship with predictability. Perfect predictability implies strict determinism, but lack of predictability does not necessarily imply lack of determinism. Limitations on predictability could alternatively be caused by factors such as a lack of information or excessive complexity. An example of this could be found by looking at a bomb dropping from the air. Through mathematics, we can predict the time the bomb will take to reach the ground, and we also know what will happen once the bomb explodes. Any small errors in prediction might arise from our not measuring some factors, such as puffs of wind or variations in air temperature along the bomb's path.

Logical determinism is the notion that all propositions, whether about the past, present or future, are either true or false. The problem of free will, in this context, is the problem of how choices can be free, given that what one does in the future is already determined as true or false in the present. This is referred to as the problem of future contingents.

Additionally, there is environmental determinism, also known as climatic or geographical determinism that holds the view that the physical environment, rather than social conditions, determines culture. Those who believe this view say that humans are strictly defined by stimulus-response (environment-behavior) and cannot deviate. Key proponents of this notion have included Ellen Churchill Semple, Ellsworth Huntington, Thomas Griffith Taylor and possibly Jared Diamond, although his status as an environmental determinist is debated.

Biological determinism is the idea that all behavior, belief, and desire are fixed by our genetic endowment. There are other theses on determinism, including *cultural determinism* and the narrower concept of *psychological determinism*. Combinations and syntheses of determinist theses, e.g. *bio-environmental determinism*, are even more common. Addiction Specialist Dr. Drew Pinski relates addiction to biological determinism: [*cite this quote*]

"Absolutely, it's a complex disorder, but it clearly has a genetic basis. In fact, in the definition of the disease, we consider genetics absolutely a crucial piece of the definition. So the definition as stated in a consensus conference that was published in the early '90s, it's a genetic disorder with a biological basis. The hallmark is the progressive use in the face of adverse consequence, and then finally denial."

Theological determinism is the thesis that there is a God who determines all that humans will do, either by knowing their actions in advance, via some form of omniscience or by decreeing their actions in advance. The problem of free will, in this context, is the problem of how our actions can be free, if there is a being who has determined them for us ahead of time.

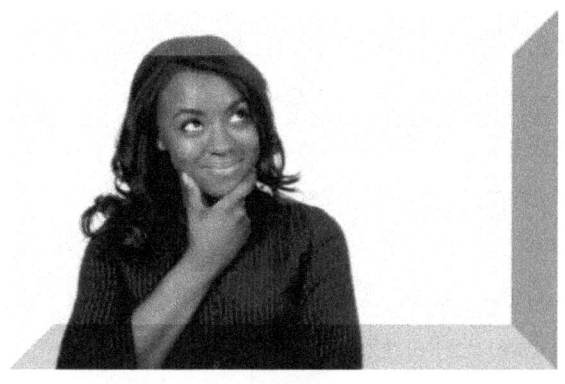

X

Philosophy of rationalism

Classical Greek rationalists

Socrates (ca 470–399B.C.E.)

Main article: Socrates

Socrates firmly believed that, before humans can understand the world, they first need to understand themselves; the only way to accomplish that is with rational thought. In order to understand what this means, one needs first to appreciate the Greek understanding of the world. Man is composed of two parts, a body and a soul. The soul itself has two principal parts, an irrational part, which is the emotions and desires, and a rational part, which is our true self. In our everyday experience, the irrational soul is drawn down into the physical body by its desires and merged with it, so that our perception of the world is limited to that delivered by the physical senses. The rational soul is beyond our conscious knowledge, but sometimes communicates via images, dreams, and other means.

The task of the philosopher is to refine and eventually extract the irrational soul from its bondage, hence the need for moral development, and then to connect with the rational soul, and so become a complete person, manifesting the higher spiritual essence of the person whilst in the physical. True rationalism is therefore not simply an intellectual process, but a shift in perception and a shift in the qualitative nature of the person. The rational soul perceives the world in a spiritual manner - it sees the Platonic Forms - the essence of what things are. To know the world in this way requires that one first know oneself as a soul, hence the requirement to 'know thyself', i.e. to know who you truly are.

Socrates did not publish or write any of his thoughts, but he was constantly in discussion with others. He would usually start by asking a rhetorical (seemingly answerable) question, to which the other would give an answer. Socrates would then continue to ask questions until all conflicts were resolved, or until the other could do nothing else but admit to not knowing the answer (which was what most of his discussions ended with). Socrates did not claim to know the answers, but that did not take away the ability to critically and rationally approach problems. His goal was to show that ultimately, our intellectual approach to the world is flawed, and we need to transcend this in order to obtain a true knowledge of what things are.

This book is dedicated to my Mom Sarah Edwards who has endured and overcome the scars that life has given her to raise six children unassisted by deadbeat dads. To my wife Carroll E. Edwards who has loved, listened and endured my scars, and my kids whom if I had not overcome would not be here today

Inspiration

My inspiration has ignited my creative

juices and I feel alive! For years, the grind

of humdrum life has sucked the once vibrant

side of me. My inspiration is oblivious to

the force exuded from her being. The aura

surrounding my inspiration is so strong an

ever present glow follows her like the heat

from pavement after a morning rain. Sweeter

than chocolate, confident in who you are,

and smoother than molasses, this is my inspiration. Some are inspired by people

they never meet, some are inspired by the

challenge that life brings. I am inspired by

you! At times there seems to be no connection

between two people and the questions arises

why do I inspire you? Because you are you!

I

was asked a question by a close friend, is

it true that you always marry your soul

mate? I said no because my soul-mate is married to someone else! **"GOD"**

Thaddeus Laverne Edwards Copyright ©2009

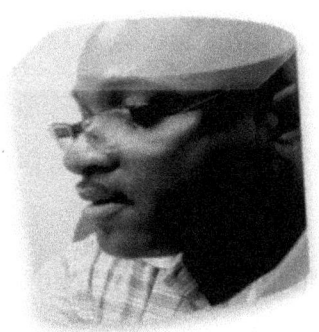

"Men supposedly rule the world, but women have great influence"

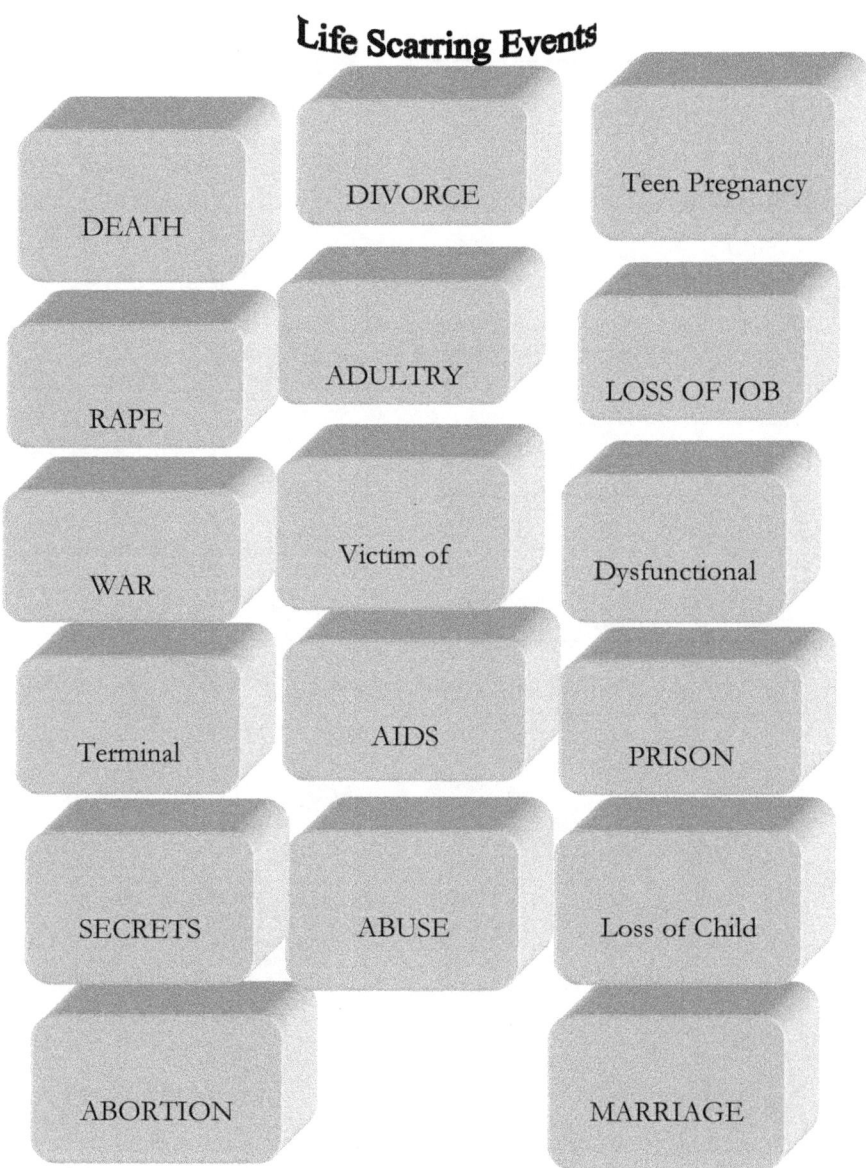

List your personal Mental and Physical scars

1. _____
2. _____
3. _____
4. _____
5. _____
6. _____
7. _____
8. _____
9. _____
10. _____

Now List the scars you have overcome

1. _____
2. _____
3. _____
4. _____
5. _____
6. _____
7. _____
8. _____
9. _____
10. _____

List your remaining scars if any

1. _____
2. _____
3. _____
4. _____
5. _____
6. _____
7. _____
8. _____
9. _____
10. _____

This list should be smaller

What are you going to do to overcome your remaining scars?

1. _____
2. _____
3. _____
4. _____
5. _____
6. _____
7. _____
8. _____
9. _____
10. _____

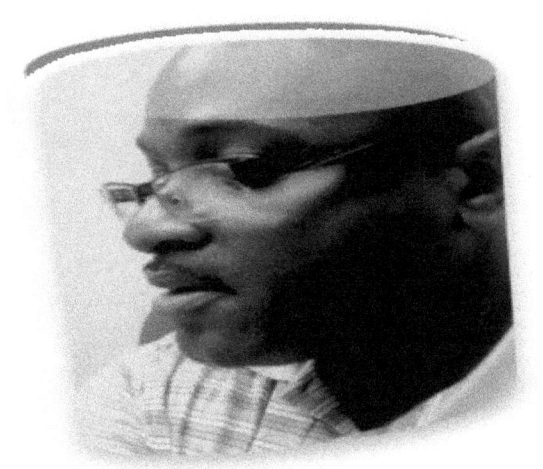

Author: Thaddeus L. Edwards

1963 Belhaven Drive

Orange Park, Florida 32065

Email: Zyardsale@gmail.com

Business number: 1.888.468.0582

Website:

http://www.zyardsale.com

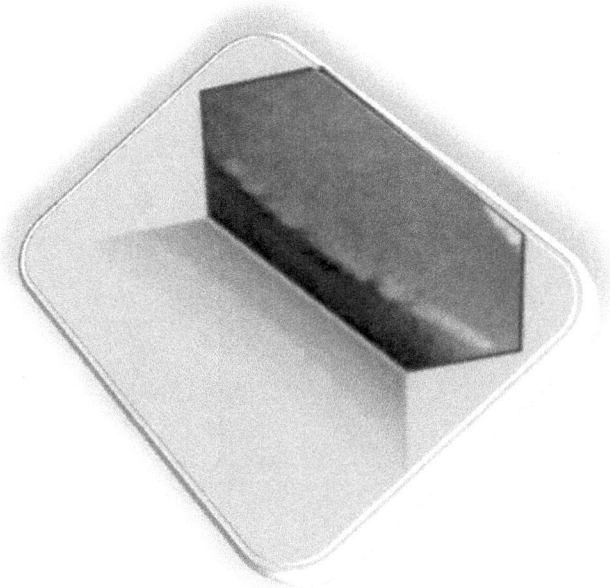

Scarred for life – The Scar from my uncle

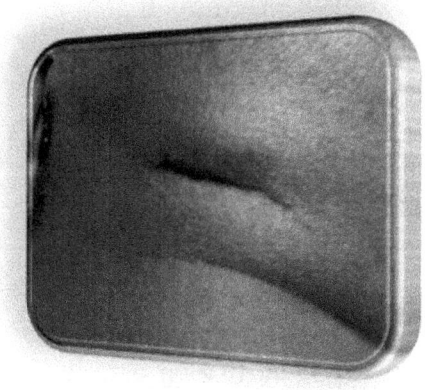

Scarred for Life – The scar from my ex-wife

Book Sponsored by:

For information regarding book signings, lectures, seminars, or order books, audio CD's, and DVD's by the author, please visit my website, call, email or write:

Thaddeus L. Edwards, Segeant First Class, USA Retired

1963 Belhaven Drive

Orange Park, Florida 32065

Email: zyardsale@gmail.com

888-468-0582

Website:

http://www.zyardsale.com

Management Consulting 904.705.9581 Zyardsale@gmail.com	**Follow us on Twitter** Twitter.com/zyardsale 904.705.9581
Speaking Engagements 904.705.9581 Zyardsale@gmail.com	**Advertising** http://www.zyardsale.com 904.705.9581
Follow us on YouTube Youtube.com/zyardsale 904.705.9581	**Family Intervention** Zyardsale@gmail.com 904.705.9581
For Book Signings Zyardsale@gmail.com 904.705.9581	**To order the book as a gift** http://www.zyardsale.com or visit LULU.com
Lectures Zyardsale@gmail.com 904.705.9581	**Seminars** Zyardsale@gmail.com 904.705.9581

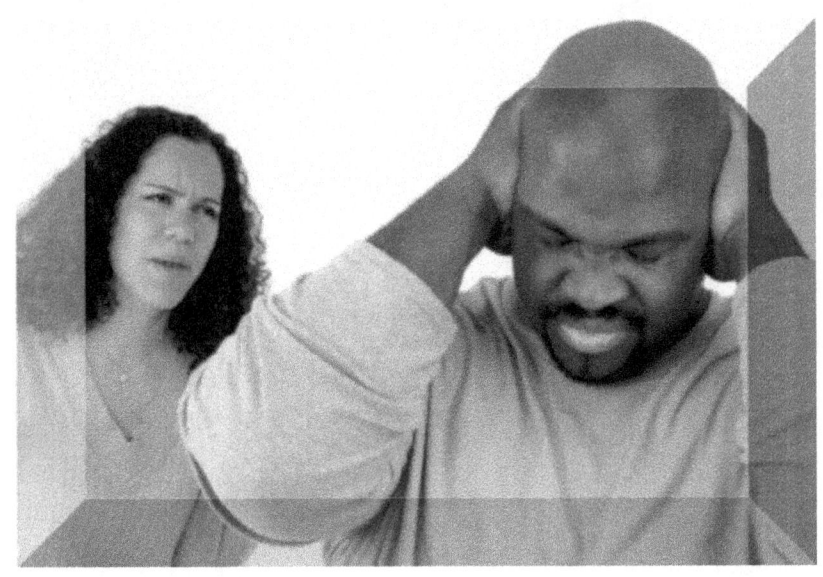

Does nagging or arguing solve the problem?

NO!

Someone needs to be the voice of reason to allow disagreements to be discussed in an peaceful manner.

A mental scar does not disappear, it only lays dormant waiting to be discussed again when adversity arises.

Find out why you get angry and learn how to use a **Power Phrase** to stop your anger before it takes control. Learn about "anger trigger behavior" and how to avoid confrontations with loved ones when angry. Best of all, you'll receive inspirational messaging to help stay motivated and in control.

Visit: Personalgrowthpath.com for help

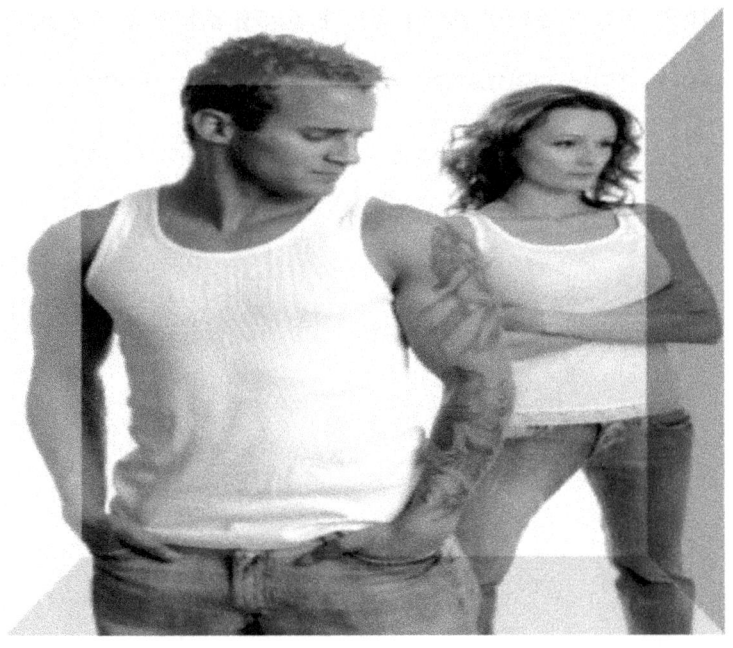

The flesh is weak! Don't allow it to scar your relationship on chance encounters.

The flesh is in constant battle with the spirit so be careful what you ask for you may get it!

For those who live according to the flesh set their minds on things according to the flesh, but those who live according to the spirit, the things of the spirit.

Romans: Chapter 8:5

Sexual addiction also is associated with risk-taking. A person with a sex addiction engages in various forms of sexual activity, despite the potential for negative and/or dangerous consequences. In addition to damaging the addict's relationships and interfering with his or her work and social life, a sexual addiction also puts the person at risk for emotional and physical injury. Visit Webmd.com

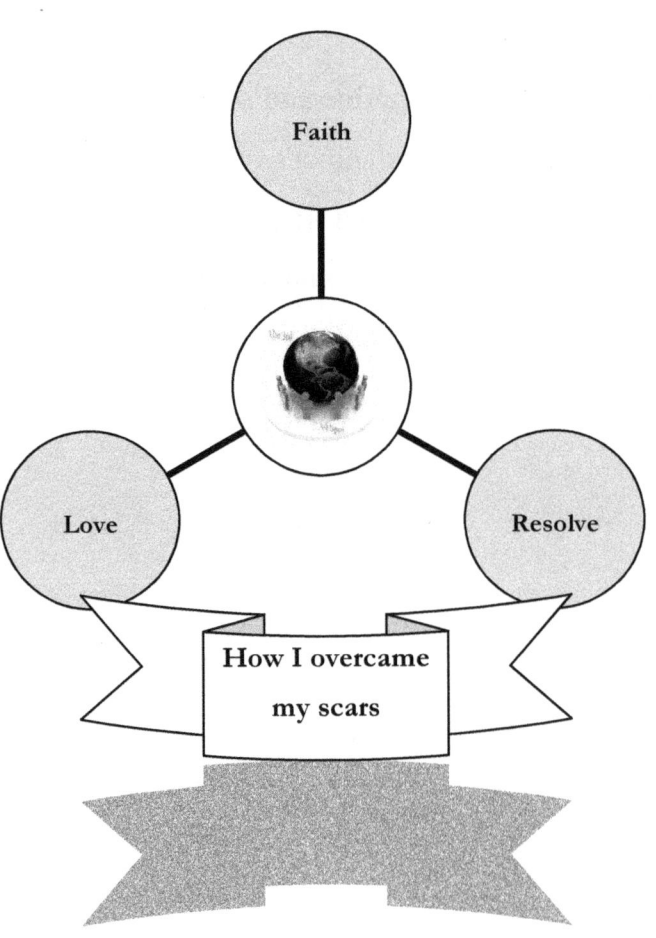

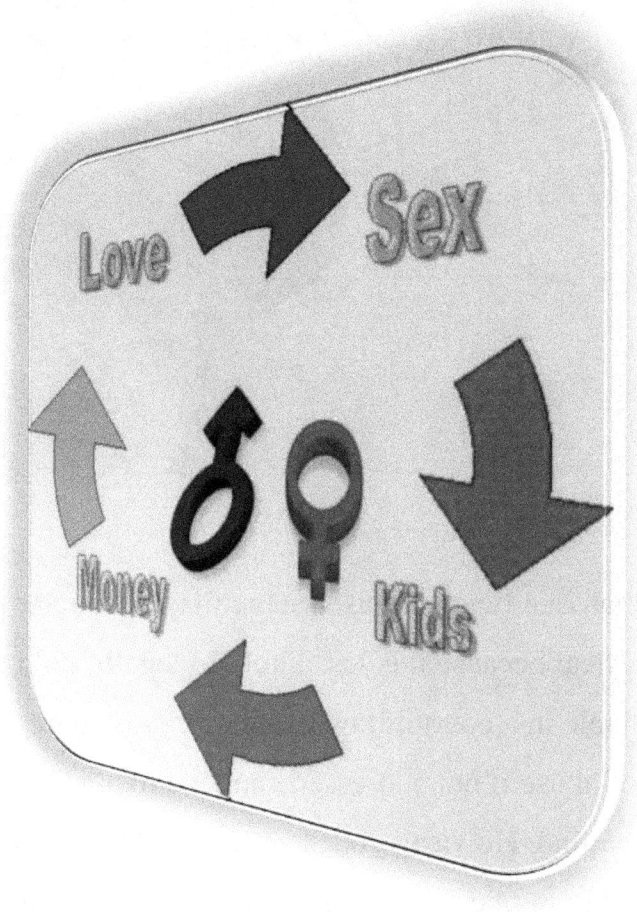

There is more than one type of abuse. Some may encounter more mental than physical because it is less likely to legally hold the mental abuser liable in a court of law. Hate crimes, and neglect are also forms of abuse if not addressed can lead to a lifetime battle within the mind. How can you stop abuse? Abuse does not rear its ugly head in public. It is a master of disguise. It hides behind smiles, seemingly unreproached behavior at work, Armani suits, and power suits. No one knows what happens behind closed doors. As an adult, you accept the responsibility to see the signs. It can only be recognized by those willing to go beneath what the eyes see, and listen to their hearts. Our society has gone straight to hell because no one wants to get involved.

Do not be that person that turns your back on those in need. You and I cannot save the planet, but my hope is that you will have a role in saving that one person. Enough is Enough!

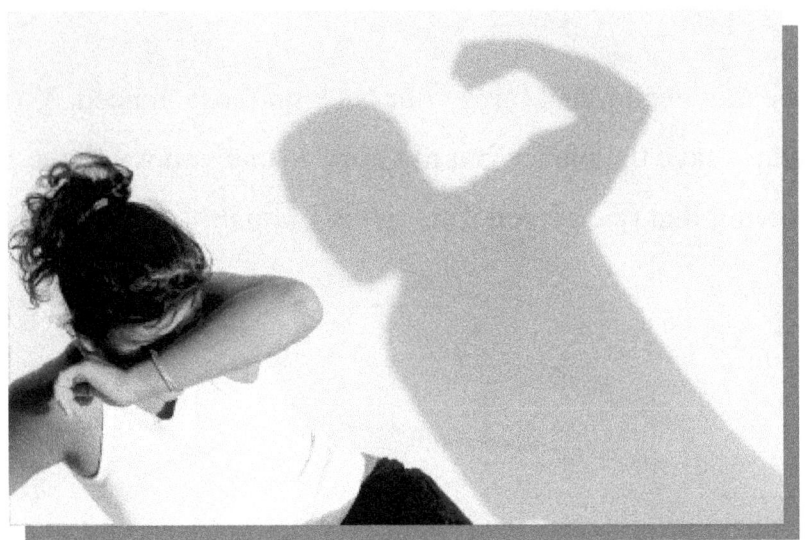

What is woman abuse?

Woman abuse is any verbal threat or physical force used to create fear and control what a woman does.

Women, don't accept what has happened before. Do something about it. At some point, you have to stop enabling his behavior. The longer you remain in these types of relationships, the deeper your scars will be. If you do not want to be scarred for life then remove yourself from this person. Women often feel that starting over would be difficult so they try to stick it out, but is your health worth perceived monetary security? Ladies if he is isolating you from your loved ones and depriving you spiritually, you need to dislodge this cancer like man and claim your freedom. Only then will you be considered a survivor of abuse. There is help, visit the site below and get out!

Womenabuseprevention.com

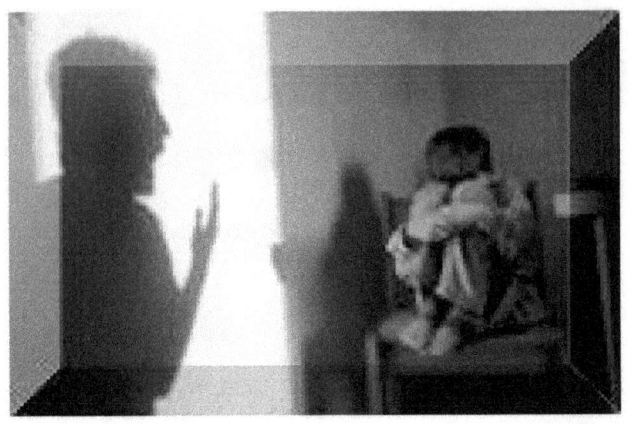

Children do not have the capacity to protect themselves. They see adults as we would view an NBA player, as a giant. A child should not have to endure the backlash of a miserable adult whose life is not going the way they want and brings it home. Be the adult; get your child out of these situations so that they will not carry this with them into their relationships. Get help today! Do not wait until it's too late to make a difference in a child's life. No child should be scarred for life.

Child Abuse Prevention Association - CAPA

    503 E. 23rd Street

    Independence, M0 64055

    816-252-8388

    Fax: 816-252-1337

    Childabuseprevention.org

Farewell Past

Obituary

The Past:

Born February 9, 1964

Place of Birth: Mobile, Alabama

Graduated from John C. Fremont High School, Los Angeles, California

Educated at: Central Texas College, University of Phoenix, and several military schools during a twenty year career.

Awards: Bronze Star Medal for combat operations in Iraq, The Meritorious Service Medal, and the Coveted Pinnacle Award

The Past loved football, golf, and music

The Past will be burried now!

Memorial contributions can be sent to you. Bury your past, that is your contribution!

The past was a wonderful experience. It taught me to mature at a faster pace. It was with me as I went through life and was a true friend. The past is being buried today, but it will not be forgotten. It is survived by love, laughter, harmony, and hope. Love was his oldest son who took on the burdens of a family mired in unhappiness. The sun is shining on love again, now that the past has gone away. Laughter resides where frowns once were. Laughter has found its way through the thick walls of jaws once wrinkled with sadness. Laughter is once again funny.

Harmony has grown so much since the past has been burried. Harmony is communicating with everyone at every opportunity in passing. Harmony is so contagious that disharmonious people transform. Hope is the youngest of the four, but it has the brightest future. Hope is open to new adventureous things now that the past has gone. The light of Hope reigns a loud voracious throng of tomorrow. Hope is alive and prepared to move on without the past. The past has served it's purpose, but it's purpose is no longer required. Farewell past, I no longer need you, I survived you, I win.

In Conclusion

Life is the problem can you solve it.

All of us have difficulty at some point in our lives that seem insurmountable. Overcoming all of our scars may or may not be attainable, but together we can minimize the effect of these scars so that living becomes enjoyable. Do you believe that you can? I believe and so should you! Life has a way of making you humble at the height of your arrogance. When it does, accept it, overcome, and don't give up.

Giving up will leave a scar within your soul. In the end, strength comes from above, and within. The will to survive the emotional and physical scars are what will define you as a human being. Will you be remembered as the one that succumbed to the scars or overcame them to lead a life to attain self-actualization? I know now that those that disparaged me only did so to make themselves feel better about their own shortcomings. Stand up, release your pain, it is only there because you allow it to be. Defeat your scars and you defeat what haunts you.

www.ingramcontent.com/pod-product-compliance
Lightning Source LLC
Chambersburg PA
CBHW032004060426
42449CB00031B/308